Stretching Made Easy Beginners Guide

Setting Up a Stretching Routine

By

Reece Klaus

Table of Contents

CHAPTER 1

Introduction

1.1 Why Stretching is Important

Stretching is a fundamental component of physical well-being and plays a crucial role in maintaining overall health and flexibility. It is an integral part of any exercise routine, sports training, or physical activity, and it offers numerous benefits that go beyond just improving flexibility. In this section, we will delve into the importance of stretching and the reasons why it should be an essential part of your daily life.

1. Enhanced Flexibility and Range of Motion: One of the primary

reasons why stretching is important is that it enhances flexibility and increases the range of motion in your joints and muscles. Regular stretching exercises gradually lengthen the muscle fibers, tendons, and connective tissues, allowing them to move more freely. Improved flexibility not only makes daily tasks easier but also helps in preventing injuries, as flexible muscles are less likely to strain or tear during physical activities.

2. Injury Prevention: Stretching can significantly reduce the risk of injuries during exercise or sports activities. When your muscles are flexible, they are less prone to sudden tears or sprains when subjected to sudden movements or forceful contractions. Stretching

helps to warm up the muscles and increase blood flow, which prepares them for the physical demands of various activities. By incorporating stretching into your pre-workout routine, you can reduce the likelihood of muscle strains, joint injuries, and other workout-related problems.

3. Improved Circulation: Stretching stimulates blood circulation throughout the body. As you stretch, blood flow to the muscle's increases, delivering oxygen and essential nutrients while removing waste products from the tissues. Improved circulation not only aids in muscle recovery but also enhances overall cardiovascular health. Proper blood flow contributes to better heart health, reduced blood pressure, and

improved endurance during physical activities.

4. Alleviation of Muscle Tension and Stress: Daily life and various activities can lead to muscle tension and stress build-up. Stretching provides an excellent way to relieve this tension and promote relaxation. When you stretch, your muscles release accumulated stress, helping you feel more relaxed and less tense. This can have a positive impact on your mental well-being, reducing anxiety and promoting a sense of calmness.

5. Enhanced Posture and Alignment: Sitting for prolonged periods, poor posture, and muscle imbalances can lead to alignment issues and postural problems. Stretching can help correct these imbalances by

lengthening tight muscles and strengthening weak ones. By addressing these postural concerns, stretching contributes to improved posture, which can alleviate back pain, neck pain, and other related discomforts.

6. Increased Athletic Performance: For athletes and individuals engaged in sports, stretching is essential to enhance performance. By increasing flexibility and range of motion, athletes can achieve optimal body mechanics and movement patterns, leading to improved athletic performance. Flexible muscles also enable athletes to generate more power and improve their agility and speed.

7. Preparing the Body for Exercise: Before engaging in any physical

activity or workout, it is essential to prepare the body properly. Stretching serves as an effective warm-up routine that prepares the muscles and joints for the upcoming exercise. Warm muscles are more pliable and less prone to injury during physical exertion. By incorporating stretching into your pre-workout routine, you can maximize the benefits of your exercise session.

8. Post-Workout Recovery: Stretching is not only beneficial before exercise but also after a workout. Engaging in post-workout stretches helps to cool down the body gradually, reducing the risk of muscle cramps and soreness. Stretching after exercise also aids in muscle recovery by promoting blood flow, which

assists in the removal of metabolic waste products that accumulate during physical activity.

stretching is a vital aspect of maintaining physical fitness, preventing injuries, and enhancing overall well-being. Its importance lies not only in improving flexibility but also in preparing the body for physical activities, alleviating muscle tension, enhancing athletic performance, and promoting post-workout recovery. Whether you are a beginner or an experienced fitness enthusiast, incorporating stretching into your daily routine can lead to a healthier and more active lifestyle. So, make stretching a priority in your life and experience the countless benefits it has to offer.

1.2 Who Should Stretch?

Stretching is beneficial for individuals of all ages and fitness levels. It is not limited to athletes or individuals engaged in intense physical activities; rather, it is a practice that can benefit everyone. Here's a breakdown of who should incorporate stretching into their routine:

1. Sedentary Individuals: People who have sedentary lifestyles, such as those who work desk jobs or spend extended periods sitting, can greatly benefit from stretching to counteract the negative effects of prolonged sitting on their muscles and posture.

2. Office Workers: Those who spend long hours at a computer or in a seated position can experience muscle tightness and discomfort.

Stretching can help alleviate these issues and improve overall well-being.

3. Older Adults: Aging can lead to a natural decline in flexibility and mobility. Stretching can be especially valuable for older adults to maintain joint health, prevent stiffness, and reduce the risk of falls.

4. Exercise Enthusiasts: Whether you engage in regular cardiovascular exercises, strength training, or sports, incorporating stretching into your fitness routine can enhance performance and reduce the risk of exercise-related injuries.

5. Recreational Athletes: People who participate in recreational sports or physical activities can benefit from stretching to improve their athletic

performance, reduce the risk of strains, and enhance overall mobility.

6. Individuals Recovering from Injuries: Stretching can be part of a rehabilitation program for individuals recovering from certain injuries. It can aid in regaining flexibility and restoring normal muscle function.

7. Pregnant Women: Prenatal stretching can help pregnant women manage discomfort, improve circulation, and maintain flexibility during pregnancy.

8. Stress Management Seekers: Stretching provides an opportunity for relaxation and mindfulness, making it suitable for individuals seeking stress relief and mental well-being.

Overall, stretching is a versatile practice suitable for individuals of all backgrounds and lifestyles. Whether you're looking to improve flexibility, prevent injuries, or simply enhance your physical and mental well-being, incorporating stretching into your daily routine can be a valuable and rewarding endeavor.

1.3 Safety Considerations

While stretching offers numerous benefits, it is essential to practice it safely to avoid potential injuries or adverse effects. Here are some important safety considerations to keep in mind when incorporating stretching into your routine:

1. Warm-up before Stretching:
    Always warm up your body before
    engaging in stretching exercises.
    Cold muscles are more prone to
    injury, so start with light aerobic
    activities like walking or jogging
    for a few minutes to increase blood
    flow and raise your body
    temperature.

2. Avoid Bouncing: Avoid bouncing
    or jerking movements during
    stretching, as this can lead to
    muscle strains or tears. Instead,
    perform stretches smoothly and
    gradually, holding the position
    without sudden movements.

3. Listen to Your Body: Pay attention
    to your body's signals during
    stretching. Stretch only to the point
    of mild tension or discomfort, not
    to the point of pain. If you feel
    pain during a stretch, stop

immediately and assess if you are doing the stretch correctly.

4. Don't Overstretch: Overstretching can cause muscle or ligament injuries. Avoid pushing your body beyond its natural range of motion, especially if you are a beginner or have not been regularly stretching.

5. Focus on Proper Form: Ensure that you are using proper form during stretching exercises. Incorrect form can lead to imbalances or strain certain muscles. If you are unsure about the correct technique, consider seeking guidance from a qualified fitness professional or physical therapist.

6. Gradual Progression: Gradually increase the intensity and duration of your stretching routine over time. Rushing into advanced

stretches can increase the risk of injury. Start with basic stretches and gradually progress as your flexibility improves.

7. Avoid Stretching Cold Muscles: Stretching cold muscles can lead to strains. Avoid static stretching (holding a stretch) before engaging in intense physical activities. Save static stretching for after your workout when your muscles are warm.

8. Include Dynamic Warm-up: Before workouts or physical activities, include dynamic warm-up exercises that mimic the movements you'll be doing. Dynamic warm-ups help prepare your body for the specific demands of your chosen activity.

9. Be Cautious with Injuries: If you have a previous injury or medical condition, consult with a healthcare professional or physical therapist before starting a stretching routine. Certain stretches may not be suitable or could exacerbate existing injuries.

10. Breathe and Relax: Remember to breathe deeply and relax while stretching. Holding your breath or tensing up can inhibit the effectiveness of the stretch and increase the risk of injury.

11. Stretch All Major Muscle Groups: Include stretches that target all major muscle groups to promote overall flexibility and prevent imbalances.

12. Stay Hydrated: Proper hydration is essential for overall health and can

contribute to muscle flexibility. Drink enough water throughout the day, including before and after stretching sessions.

13. Stretch on a Stable Surface: Perform stretching exercises on a stable and even surface to reduce the risk of slips or falls.

By following these safety considerations, you can make stretching a safe and beneficial part of your daily routine. Remember to be patient with your progress, and if you experience any pain or discomfort during stretching, consult with a healthcare professional or fitness expert to address any concerns. Safe and proper stretching can lead to improved flexibility, reduced risk of injuries, and enhanced overall physical well-being.

CHAPTER 2

Understanding the Basics of Stretching

2.1 Different Types of Stretching

Stretching is not a one-size-fits-all practice, as there are various techniques that target different muscle groups and serve different purposes. Understanding the different types of stretching can help you tailor your stretching routine to meet your specific needs and goals. Here are the four main types of stretching:

2.1.1 Static Stretching

Static stretching is one of the most common and straightforward forms of stretching. It involves holding a stretch in a fixed position for a certain amount of time, typically between 15 to 60 seconds. The goal of static stretching is to gradually lengthen the muscle and improve its flexibility over time. This type of stretching is best performed after a workout or physical activity when the muscles are warm and more pliable.

During static stretching, you should focus on relaxing the muscles being stretched and avoid any bouncing or jerking movements. Instead, ease into the stretch until you feel a gentle tension in the muscle, and then hold the position without causing pain. Common static stretches include hamstring stretches, quadriceps stretches, and shoulder stretches.

2.1.2 Dynamic Stretching

Dynamic stretching involves active movements that take the muscles and joints through a full range of motion. Unlike static stretching, dynamic stretching is more suitable as a warm-up before physical activities or workouts. It helps increase blood flow, heart rate, and body temperature, preparing the muscles and joints for more intense movements.

Dynamic stretching can involve leg swings, arm circles, walking lunges, or other controlled movements that mimic the motions you'll be doing during your chosen activity. The emphasis is on continuous movement and gradually increasing the range of motion with each repetition.

2.1.3 Proprioceptive Neuromuscular Facilitation (PNF) Stretching

PNF stretching is an advanced stretching technique that involves a combination of stretching and muscle contraction. It is often used in physical therapy and sports rehabilitation settings. PNF stretching is highly effective for increasing flexibility and is typically performed with a partner or a trained professional.

The process usually begins with a static stretch, where the muscle is elongated to its end range. Then, the individual contracts the muscle against resistance (usually provided by a partner) for about 5-10 seconds. After the contraction, the muscle is relaxed, and the partner helps to stretch it further. This cycle is repeated for a few rounds, gradually increasing the range of motion with each contraction-relaxation phase.

2.1.4 Ballistic Stretching

Ballistic stretching involves using repetitive, bouncing movements to push the muscles beyond their normal range of motion. While it was once popular among athletes, it is now generally considered less safe than other stretching methods, as it can lead to muscle strains and injuries.

The bouncing movements in ballistic stretching can cause the muscles to contract suddenly, potentially causing overstretching and tearing. Therefore, it is generally not recommended, and most fitness experts advise against incorporating ballistic stretching into your routine.

understanding the different types of stretching allows you to choose the most appropriate stretching techniques based on your specific needs and goals. Static stretching is great for increasing overall flexibility and is best performed after a workout. Dynamic stretching is ideal for warming up before physical activities. PNF stretching is an advanced technique that can improve flexibility when performed with a partner. However, ballistic stretching is discouraged due to its potential risk of injury. Remember to consult with a fitness professional or physical therapist if you have any questions about which type of stretching is suitable for you.

2.2 When to Stretch: Pre-Workout vs. Post-Workout

The timing of stretching can significantly impact its effectiveness and your overall workout performance. Whether you should stretch before or after a workout depends on your goals and the type of stretching you plan to do. Here's a breakdown of when to stretch:

Pre-Workout Stretching: Pre-workout stretching is best performed as part of your warm-up routine. The primary goal of pre-workout stretching is to prepare the muscles and joints for the upcoming physical activity. When you stretch before a workout, it helps to increase blood flow to the muscles, raise your body temperature, and gradually improve flexibility.

It is important to note that static stretching, where you hold stretches for an extended period, is not recommended as the sole warm-up before intense activities. Static stretching can temporarily reduce muscle strength and power, which can negatively impact your workout performance and increase the risk of injury.

Instead, opt for dynamic stretching during your pre-workout warm-up. Dynamic stretches involve active movements that mimic the motions you'll be doing during your workout. This can include leg swings, arm circles, high knees, or walking lunges. Dynamic stretching helps activate the muscles, improve joint mobility, and get your body ready for the demands of the exercise ahead.

Post-Workout Stretching: Post-workout stretching is performed after your workout or physical activity. The primary goal of post-workout stretching is to aid in muscle recovery, reduce muscle soreness, and maintain or improve flexibility.

Static stretching is most suitable for post-workout sessions. Holding static stretches after a workout can help relax the muscles and improve their flexibility. Since the muscles are already warm from the exercise, static stretching is more effective and less likely to cause injury compared to pre-workout static stretching.

Post-workout stretching can also help reduce muscle tightness and improve blood circulation, which aids in the removal of metabolic waste products that accumulate during exercise. By incorporating post-workout stretching into your routine, you can promote muscle recovery and enhance overall flexibility over time.

2.3 How Long to Hold Stretches

The duration for which you should hold stretches depends on the type of stretching you are performing. Here are general guidelines for how long to hold stretches:

Static Stretching: For static stretches, the commonly recommended duration is between 15 to 60 seconds per stretch. Holding a static stretch for at least 15 seconds allows the muscles to gradually lengthen and increase flexibility. You can opt to hold the stretch for longer, up to 60 seconds, for a more substantial effect.

However, avoid holding stretches for too long, as this can lead to muscle fatigue or overstretching.

Dynamic Stretching: Dynamic stretches involve continuous movements, so they are not held in a fixed position like static stretches. Aim for about 10 to 15 repetitions for each dynamic stretch. The focus should be on controlled and smooth movements, gradually increasing the range of motion with each repetition.

PNF Stretching: For PNF stretching, follow the pattern of contracting the muscle against resistance for 5-10 seconds, then relaxing and stretching it further. Repeat this cycle for a few rounds, progressively increasing the stretch with each cycle.

Ballistic Stretching: As mentioned earlier, ballistic stretching is generally discouraged due to its potential risk of injury. Therefore, the duration is not applicable for this type of stretching.

Remember that stretching should never cause pain. If you feel pain during a stretch, ease off the tension and avoid pushing yourself too hard. Consistency is key to improving flexibility, so incorporate stretching into your routine regularly, both before and after workouts, to enjoy its full benefits. If you have any specific concerns or medical conditions, consider consulting with a fitness professional or physical therapist for personalized stretching recommendations.

CHAPTER 3

Setting Up a Stretching Routine

3.1 Assessing Your Flexibility

Before establishing a stretching routine, it's essential to assess your current level of flexibility. Assessing your flexibility will help you identify areas that need improvement and determine the most appropriate stretches for your needs. Here are some steps to assess your flexibility:

1. Warm-Up: Start with a light warm-up to increase blood flow to your muscles and prepare them for stretching. You can do some light

cardiovascular exercises like brisk walking, cycling, or jogging for 5-10 minutes.

2. Neck and Shoulders: Gently tilt your head forward, backward, and sideways to assess the range of motion in your neck. For your shoulders, try reaching one arm across your chest and using the other hand to press gently on your forearm, feeling the stretch in your shoulder and upper arm. Repeat on the other side.

3. Arms and Chest: Stretch your arms overhead and behind your back to assess the flexibility of your shoulders and chest muscles.

4. Back and Core: Perform seated or standing forward bends to assess the flexibility of your lower back and hamstrings. You can also try a

cat-cow stretch on all fours to evaluate the flexibility of your spine.

5. Hips and Legs: Test the flexibility of your hips and legs with exercises like lunges, seated or standing leg raises, and hip flexor stretches.

6. Ankles and Calves: Sit or stand with your legs extended and point and flex your feet to assess the range of motion in your ankles and calves.

7. Note Your Range of Motion: As you perform each stretch, pay attention to how far you can comfortably move your joints and muscles. Take note of any areas that feel particularly tight or restricted.

8. Use a Flexibility Test: There are specific flexibility tests designed to measure the range of motion in various joints and muscle groups. Examples include the sit-and-reach test for hamstring flexibility and the shoulder flexion test for shoulder flexibility.

9. Consider Limitations: Take into account any previous injuries or medical conditions that may affect your flexibility. Certain conditions may require modifications to your stretching routine or the need to consult with a healthcare professional or physical therapist.

10. Document Your Findings: Keep a record of your flexibility assessment, noting any improvements over time. This will help you track your progress and

adjust your stretching routine accordingly.

Based on your flexibility assessment, you can tailor your stretching routine to focus on areas that need improvement. Incorporate a mix of static and dynamic stretches into your routine, targeting different muscle groups and joints. Gradually increase the intensity and duration of your stretches as your flexibility improves. Remember to always warm up before stretching and avoid overstretching or pushing yourself into painful positions. With consistency and proper technique, regular stretching can lead to improved flexibility and overall physical well-being.

3.2 Designing Your Stretching Program

Creating a well-rounded stretching program involves considering warm-up exercises, targeted muscle groups, and cool-down stretches. A comprehensive program can help improve flexibility, reduce the risk of injuries, and enhance overall physical performance. Here's how to design an effective stretching routine:

3.2.1 Warm-up Exercises

Before diving into stretching, warm up your body with some light aerobic activities to increase blood flow, elevate your heart rate, and raise your body temperature. Warm-up exercises should be dynamic in nature, involving active movements that mimic the motions you'll be doing during your workout or physical activity. Aim to spend about 5-10 minutes on your warm-up. Here are some warm-up exercises you can include:

1. Arm Circles: Stand with your feet shoulder-width apart and extend your arms straight out to the sides. Make circular motions with your arms, gradually increasing the circle's size. After a few rotations, switch directions.

2. Leg Swings: Hold onto a sturdy object for support and swing one leg forward and backward, keeping it straight. Repeat on the other leg. Then, swing each leg sideways, crossing it in front of your body and then behind.

3. Hip Rotations: Stand with your hands on your hips and rotate your hips in a circular motion, first in one direction and then the other.

4. High Knees: Stand tall and march in place, lifting your knees as high as possible while swinging your arms to mimic a running motion.

5. Walking Lunges: Take forward lunging steps, keeping your back straight and your front knee aligned with your ankle. Alternate between left and right legs

3.2.2 Targeted Muscle Groups

Design your stretching program to target all major muscle groups. Include a mix of static and dynamic stretches to promote overall flexibility. Focus on the areas you identified during your flexibility assessment as well as those commonly affected by your daily activities or workouts. Here are some examples of stretches for various muscle groups:

1. Neck and Shoulders: Neck stretches, shoulder rolls, and shoulder stretches.

2. Arms and Chest: Triceps stretches, chest openers, and bicep stretches.

3. Back and Core: Cat-cow stretches, seated or standing forward bends, and spinal twists.

4. Hips and Legs: Hip flexor stretches, quad stretches, hamstring stretches, calf stretches, and inner thigh stretches.

5. Ankles and Calves: Ankle circles, calf raises, and Achilles tendon stretches.

3.2.3 Cool-Down Stretches

After completing your workout or physical activity, it's time for cool-down stretches to help your body gradually return to a state of rest. Cool-down stretches should be static and held for about 15 to 30 seconds per stretch. This can help reduce muscle soreness, increase flexibility, and promote relaxation. Here are some cool-down stretches you can include:

1. Seated Forward Bend: Sit with your legs extended in front of you and reach for your toes or shins, aiming to keep your back straight.

2. Child's Pose: Kneel on the floor and sit back on your heels, then reach your arms forward as far as possible while lowering your chest toward the floor.

3. Quadriceps Stretch: Stand on one leg, bend your knee, and grab your ankle with the corresponding hand, pulling your heel toward your glutes.

4. Pigeon Pose: Sit with one knee bent in front of you and the other leg extended straight back. Lean forward to feel a stretch in the hip of the extended leg.

5. Standing Forward Bend: Stand with your feet hip-width apart and bend forward at your hips, reaching for the floor or your shins. Allow your head and neck to relax.

6. Chest Opener: Interlace your fingers behind your back and straighten your arms while lifting your chest and opening your shoulders.

Breathe deeply and focus on relaxing during your cool-down stretches. Gradually ease into each stretch and avoid any bouncing or sudden movements.

To create a balanced stretching routine, consider the time you have available and your specific fitness goals. For a comprehensive stretching program, allocate about 15-30 minutes for your routine, including warm-up and cool-down. Be consistent with your stretching program, performing it at least three times a week, if not daily, to maximize its benefits. If you are new to stretching or have any medical conditions, consult with a fitness professional or physical therapist to ensure you design a safe and effective stretching routine that meets your individual needs.

CHAPTER 4

Step-by-Step Stretching Exercises

4.1 Neck and Shoulders

Before starting the neck and shoulder stretches, sit or stand in a comfortable position with good posture. Avoid any sudden or jerky movements during these stretches. Hold each stretch for about 15-30 seconds and repeat on both sides if applicable. If you experience any pain or discomfort, stop the stretch immediately.

1. Neck Side Stretch:

- Sit or stand tall with your shoulders relaxed.

- Slowly tilt your head to one side, bringing your ear toward your shoulder.

- Hold the stretch on each side, feeling a gentle stretch along the side of your neck.

- Repeat on the other side.

2. Neck Forward and Backward Stretch:

- Sit or stand tall with your shoulders relaxed.

- Gently lower your chin toward your chest to stretch the back of your neck.

- Slowly lift your head back up and look up toward the ceiling to stretch the front of your neck.

- Repeat this forward and backward movement, maintaining control and avoiding excessive strain.

3. Neck Rotation:

- Sit or stand tall with your shoulders relaxed.

- Turn your head to one side, bringing your chin over your shoulder.

- Hold the stretch, feeling a gentle stretch in the side of your neck.

- Return to the center and repeat on the other side.

4. Shoulder Rolls:

- Stand with your feet shoulder-width apart and your arms hanging at your sides.

- Roll your shoulders forward in a circular motion, making big circles with your shoulders.

- After a few rotations, roll your shoulders backward in the same circular motion.

4.2 Arms and Chest

Perform these arm and chest stretches in a controlled manner, avoiding any sudden or forceful movements. Hold each stretch for about 15-30 seconds, and repeat if desired.

1. Triceps Stretch:

- Raise one arm overhead and bend your elbow, reaching your hand down your back.

- Use your opposite hand to gently press on the bent elbow, feeling a stretch along the back of your arm.

- Repeat on the other arm.

2. Chest Opener:

- Stand tall with your feet hip-width apart.

- Interlace your fingers behind your back and straighten your arms.

- Lift your chest and open your shoulders as you press your arms slightly backward.

- Hold the stretch and breathe deeply.

3. Shoulder Cross Stretch:

- Bring one arm across your chest at shoulder height.

- Use your opposite hand to gently pull the extended arm closer to your chest.

- Feel the stretch in the back of your shoulder.

- Repeat on the other arm.

4. Bicep Stretch:

- Stand with your feet hip-width apart.

- Extend one arm in front of you with your palm facing up.

- Use your opposite hand to gently pull back on your fingers, feeling a stretch in your bicep.

- Repeat on the other arm.

Maintain proper posture and avoid any pain or discomfort during these stretches. Incorporate these neck and shoulder stretches, along with the arms and chest stretches, into your stretching routine to enhance flexibility and reduce tension in these areas. If you have any specific neck, shoulder, or arm issues, consider consulting with a healthcare professional or physical therapist before performing these stretches.

4.3 Back and Core

When performing back and core stretches, ensure that you maintain proper form and control. Hold each stretch for about 15-30 seconds and repeat if desired. Avoid any bouncing or jerking movements during these stretches. If you experience any pain or discomfort, stop the stretch immediately.

1. Cat-Cow Stretch:

- Start on your hands and knees in a tabletop position.

- Inhale as you arch your back, lifting your head and tailbone towards the ceiling (Cow Pose).

- Exhale as you round your back, tucking your chin and tailbone (Cat Pose).

- Flow smoothly between Cat and Cow poses, focusing on your breath.

2. Child's Pose:

- Begin on your hands and knees in a tabletop position.

- Sit back on your heels, extending your arms forward and lowering your chest towards the floor.

- Relax your forehead on the mat or
  floor and feel a gentle stretch in
  your lower back and hips.

3. Seated Forward Bend:

- Sit with your legs extended in
  front of you.

- Inhale as you lengthen your spine,
  and then exhale as you hinge at
  your hips to reach forward towards
  your toes or shins.

- Keep your back straight and avoid
  rounding your shoulders.

- Hold the stretch, feeling a gentle
  stretch in your lower back and
  hamstrings.

4. Child's Pose with Side Reach:

- Start in a Child's Pose position
  (sitting back on your heels, arms
  extended forward).

- Walk your hands to one side, feeling a stretch along the side of your body.

- Hold the stretch and breathe deeply, then repeat on the other side.

4.4 Legs and Hips

Perform these leg and hip stretches with control and ease. Hold each stretch for about 15-30 seconds, and repeat on both sides if applicable. Avoid pushing yourself too hard and listen to your body.

1. Hip Flexor Stretch:

- Kneel on one knee, with the other leg bent at a 90-degree angle in front of you.

- Lean forward slightly, feeling a stretch in the front of your hip on the kneeling leg.

- To deepen the stretch, lift your arm on the same side as the kneeling leg, reaching towards the ceiling.

2. Quadriceps Stretch:

- Stand tall and bend one knee, bringing your heel towards your glutes.

- Hold your foot with your hand on the same side, feeling a stretch in the front of your thigh.

- Keep your knees close together and avoid arching your lower back.

3. Hamstring Stretch:

- Sit on the floor with one leg extended straight in front of you.

- Bend the other leg and place the sole of your foot against your inner thigh.

- Lean forward from your hips, reaching towards your extended foot.

- Keep your back straight and avoid rounding your shoulders.

4. Inner Thigh Stretch:

- Sit tall with your legs extended to the sides.

- Gently lean forward, walking your hands towards one foot.

- Feel a stretch along the inner thigh of the extended leg.

- Repeat on the other side.

Incorporate these back and core stretches, along with the legs and hips stretches, into your stretching routine to promote flexibility and reduce muscle tension in these areas. As with any stretching routine, listen to your body and avoid pushing yourself beyond your limits. If you have any specific back, core, leg, or hip issues, consider consulting with a healthcare professional or physical therapist before performing these stretches.

4.5 Flexibility for Everyday Activities

Flexibility is not only beneficial for athletic performance and workouts but also plays a crucial role in improving your ability to perform everyday activities with ease and comfort. Incorporating stretches that target muscles commonly used in daily life can enhance your functional flexibility. Here are some stretches that can help improve flexibility for everyday activities:

1. Hip Opener:

- Sit on the edge of a chair or bench with your feet flat on the floor.

- Cross one ankle over the opposite knee, creating a figure-four shape with your legs.

- Gently press down on the raised knee to feel a stretch in the hip and glute area.

- Repeat on the other side.

2. Standing Calf Stretch:

- Stand facing a wall with your hands pressed against it at shoulder height.

- Step one foot back, keeping it straight and the heel on the floor.

- Bend the front knee slightly, feeling a stretch in the calf of the back leg.

- Repeat on the other side.

3. Wrist and Forearm Stretch:

- Extend one arm straight in front of you with your palm facing down.

- Use the other hand to gently pull the fingers of the extended hand towards you.

- Feel a stretch in the wrist and forearm.

- Repeat on the other hand.

4. Lower Back Twist:

- Sit on a chair with your feet flat on the floor.

- Rotate your upper body to one side, placing one hand on the back of the chair and the other hand on the armrest or seat.

- Gently twist your torso, feeling a stretch in your lower back and oblique muscles.

- Repeat on the other side.

5. Shoulder Stretch:

- Stand tall and reach one arm across your chest at shoulder height.

- Use the opposite hand to gently pull the extended arm towards your body.

- Feel a stretch in the shoulder and upper arm.

- Repeat on the other side.

6. Hamstring Stretch (Seated):

- Sit on the edge of a chair with your feet flat on the floor.

- Extend one leg straight in front of you, keeping the knee slightly bent.

- Lean forward at your hips, reaching towards your toes or shin.

- Feel a stretch in the hamstring of the extended leg.

- Repeat on the other leg.

7. Neck Stretch:

- Sit or stand tall with your shoulders relaxed.

- Tilt your head to one side, bringing your ear towards your shoulder.

- Hold the stretch to feel a gentle stretch along the side of your neck.

- Repeat on the other side.

Doing these everyday flexibility stretches into your daily routine, you can improve your mobility and range of motion, making everyday tasks more comfortable and efficient. As with any stretching program, perform these stretches slowly and gently, and avoid any movements that cause pain. If you have any specific concerns or medical conditions, consider consulting with a healthcare professional or physical therapist to customize a flexibility routine that suits your individual needs.

CHAPTER 5

Tips for Effective Stretching

5.1 Breathing Techniques during Stretching

Breathing is an essential aspect of effective stretching. Proper breathing techniques can enhance the benefits of stretching and help you relax into the stretches more effectively. Here are some tips for incorporating proper breathing into your stretching routine:

1. Breathe Deeply: Take slow, deep breaths throughout each stretch. Inhale deeply through your nose, expanding your diaphragm and

filling your lungs with air. Exhale slowly through your mouth, releasing tension and stress.

2. Stay Relaxed: Keep your muscles and body relaxed as you stretch. Avoid holding your breath or tensing up during the stretches. Instead, focus on maintaining a calm and steady breath.

3. Coordinate Breathing with Movement: For dynamic stretches, coordinate your breathing with the movement. Inhale as you prepare for the stretch, and exhale as you move into the stretch. Inhale again as you return to the starting position.

4. Breathe into the Stretch: As you hold a static stretch, imagine breathing into the specific area being stretched. Visualize your

breath flowing to the targeted muscle group, allowing it to relax and release tension.

5. Use Breath to Enhance Flexibility: During static stretches, take advantage of your exhales to gently deepen the stretch. As you exhale, try to relax further into the stretch without forcing it.

6. Avoid Breath-Holding: Holding your breath while stretching can create tension and restrict your range of motion. It can also raise your blood pressure, which is not conducive to relaxation.

7. Maintain a Steady Rhythm: Establish a steady breathing rhythm during your stretching routine. Consistency in your breath can help you maintain focus and

create a meditative aspect to your stretching practice.

8. Stay Mindful: Use your breath as an anchor to stay present and mindful during stretching. Focus on the sensation of the stretch and the rhythm of your breath, bringing your attention back if your mind starts to wander.

9. Listen to Your Body: Pay attention to how your body responds to each stretch. If you feel discomfort or pain, back off and adjust the stretch as needed. Your breath can be a valuable indicator of whether you are pushing too hard or holding the stretch safely.

By incorporating proper breathing techniques into your stretching routine, you can enhance relaxation, improve flexibility, and reduce the risk of injury. Breathing mindfully during stretching also helps create a mind-body connection, promoting a sense of calmness and well-being. Remember to be patient with yourself and enjoy the process of stretching, making it a mindful and rejuvenating practice.

5.2 Maintaining Proper Posture

Maintaining proper posture during stretching is crucial for ensuring effective and safe stretches. Proper posture allows you to target the intended muscles more effectively and reduces the risk of strain or injury. Here are some tips for maintaining proper posture during stretching:

1. Align Your Body: Start each stretch with proper alignment. Stand tall or sit up straight, ensuring that your head, shoulders, and hips are in a straight line. Avoid slouching or arching your back excessively.

2. Engage Your Core: Throughout each stretch, engage your core muscles to stabilize your spine and pelvis. A strong core provides a stable foundation for safe stretching and prevents excessive strain on your lower back.

3. Relax Your Shoulders: Keep your shoulders relaxed and away from your ears. Tension in the shoulders can hinder the effectiveness of the stretch and lead to unnecessary strain.

4. Maintain a Neutral Spine: For most stretches, maintain a neutral spine without rounding or overarching your back. This applies to standing, seated, and lying positions.

5. Pay Attention to Hips and Pelvis: Keep your hips and pelvis level and avoid tilting or twisting them during stretches. Proper alignment of the pelvis ensures that the stretch targets the intended muscle groups effectively.

6. Avoid Overstretching: Never force your body into a position that feels uncomfortable or painful. Stretch only to the point of mild tension and listen to your body's limits. Pushing too hard can lead to injury.

7. Use Props if Needed: Props like yoga blocks, straps, or cushions can help you maintain proper posture during certain stretches. They can provide support and assistance in achieving the correct alignment.

8. Focus on the Breath: Breathing deeply and mindfully can aid in maintaining proper posture. Proper breathing encourages relaxation and helps you stay centered during the stretches.

9. Modify Stretches as Necessary: If you find it challenging to maintain proper posture in a particular stretch, consider modifying the position or using a variation that suits your flexibility level and limitations.

10. Practice Regularly: Consistent practice of stretching helps improve flexibility and posture over time. Regular stretching sessions create muscle memory, making it easier to maintain proper posture throughout the day.

11. Seek Professional Guidance: If you are unsure about maintaining proper posture during certain stretches or have specific concerns, consider seeking guidance from a fitness professional or physical therapist.

By paying attention to proper posture during stretching, you can maximize the benefits of each stretch and prevent discomfort or injury. Incorporate these posture tips into your stretching routine to improve flexibility, reduce muscle tension, and enhance overall well-being.

5.3 Avoiding Common Mistakes

Avoiding common mistakes during stretching is essential to prevent injuries and ensure that you get the most out of your stretching routine. Here are some common mistakes to watch out for and how to avoid them:

1. Bouncing or Jerking Movements: Avoid using bouncing or jerking movements during stretching, as this can lead to muscle strains or tears. Instead, perform stretches smoothly and gradually, holding the position without sudden movements.

2. Overstretching: Avoid pushing your body beyond its natural range of motion, especially if you are a beginner or have not been regularly stretching.

Overstretching can lead to injuries, so always stretch to the point of mild tension, not pain.

3. Holding Your Breath: Holding your breath during stretching can cause tension and restrict your range of motion. Remember to breathe deeply and rhythmically throughout each stretch to promote relaxation and focus.

4. Ignoring Pain: Stretching should not cause pain. If you feel pain during a stretch, stop immediately and assess if you are doing the stretch correctly. Modify the stretch or seek guidance from a professional if needed.

5. Skipping the Warm-Up: Always warm up your body before engaging in stretching exercises. Cold muscles are more prone to

injury, so start with light aerobic activities like walking or jogging for a few minutes to increase blood flow and raise your body temperature.

6. Neglecting Cool-Down Stretches: After your workout or physical activity, make sure to include cool-down stretches to help your body gradually return to a state of rest. Cool-down stretches aid in muscle recovery and reduce muscle soreness.

7. Rushing Through Stretches: Take your time during each stretch and hold them for an adequate amount of time (typically 15-30 seconds). Rushing through stretches may limit their effectiveness.

8. Focusing on Only One Muscle Group: Create a balanced

stretching routine that targets all major muscle groups. Neglecting certain muscle groups can lead to imbalances and potential issues down the line.

9. Forgetting to Hydrate: Proper hydration is crucial for overall health and can contribute to muscle flexibility. Drink enough water throughout the day, including before and after stretching sessions.

10. Not Listening to Your Body: Pay attention to your body's signals during stretching. If a stretch doesn't feel right, modify it or skip it altogether. Listen to your body's limits and adjust your stretching routine accordingly.

11. Neglecting Rest Days: Allow your body time to rest and recover

between stretching sessions. Overstretching or stretching on consecutive days without rest can lead to fatigue and potential injuries.

Being mindful of these common mistakes, you can make your stretching routine safer, more effective, and enjoyable. Remember that stretching is a gradual process, and consistency is key to improving flexibility and preventing injuries. If you have specific concerns or medical conditions, consider consulting with a fitness professional or physical therapist for personalized stretching guidance.

5.4 Overcoming Plateaus and Challenges

Overcoming plateaus and challenges in your stretching routine is a natural part of the process, and it's essential not to get discouraged. Here are some strategies to help you break through plateaus and address challenges in your stretching journey:

1. Patience and Consistency: Understand that progress in flexibility takes time. Be patient with yourself and stay consistent with your stretching routine. Even small improvements over time can lead to significant gains in flexibility.

2. Gradual Progression: Gradually increase the intensity and duration of your stretches as your flexibility improves. Push yourself slightly

beyond your comfort zone, but
avoid overstretching to prevent
injuries.

3. Set Realistic Goals: Set achievable
    and realistic goals for your
    stretching routine. Having clear
    and attainable targets can help you
    stay motivated and focused on
    your progress.

4. Vary Your Stretches: Incorporate a
    variety of stretching exercises into
    your routine to target different
    muscle groups and prevent
    monotony. Trying new stretches
    can keep your practice engaging
    and challenging.

5. Use Props and Accessories: Yoga
    blocks, straps, and foam rollers can
    assist you in achieving deeper
    stretches or modifying poses to

suit your current level of
flexibility.

6. Active Isolated Stretching:
    Consider incorporating active
    isolated stretching (AIS)
    techniques into your routine. AIS
    involves holding a stretch for only
    1-2 seconds and repeating it
    several times. This method can
    help improve flexibility without
    causing the protective stretch
    reflex.

7. PNF Stretching: Explore
    proprioceptive neuromuscular
    facilitation (PNF) stretching
    techniques, which involve a
    combination of stretching and
    muscle contractions. PNF
    stretching can help override the
    body's resistance to stretching and
    enhance flexibility.

8. Cross-Train: Engage in other physical activities that complement your stretching routine, such as yoga, Pilates, or dance. Cross-training can provide different challenges and help enhance overall flexibility.

9. Rest and Recovery: Allow your body time to rest and recover between stretching sessions. Overtraining can lead to fatigue and hinder progress. Adequate rest is essential for muscle recovery and growth.

10. Address Specific Weaknesses: Identify any specific muscle groups or areas where you are facing challenges and tailor your stretching routine to focus on improving those areas.

11. Seek Professional Guidance: If
    you feel stuck or face specific
    challenges, consider seeking
    guidance from a fitness
    professional, physical therapist, or
    experienced yoga instructor. They
    can provide personalized advice
    and adjustments to help you
    overcome plateaus.

12. Mindfulness and Visualization:
    During stretching, focus on being
    present and mindful of your body's
    sensations. Visualization
    techniques can also be helpful;
    imagine your muscles becoming
    more flexible and imagine yourself
    achieving your stretching goals.

Each person's flexibility journey is
unique, and progress may vary from
one individual to another. Celebrate
your achievements, no matter how
small, and keep a positive attitude

towards your stretching practice. With dedication, consistency, and an open mind, you can overcome plateaus and challenges, reaching new levels of flexibility and overall well-being.

CHAPTER 6

Incorporating Stretching into Your Fitness Routine

6.1 Combining Stretching with Cardiovascular Exercise

Incorporating stretching into your fitness routine is an excellent way to enhance your overall flexibility, prevent injuries, and improve performance. When combined with cardiovascular exercise, stretching can help warm up your muscles before the main workout, increase blood flow to the muscles, and aid in post-workout recovery. Here's how to effectively combine stretching with cardiovascular exercise in your fitness routine:

1. Warm-up with Dynamic Stretches: Before starting your cardiovascular workout, perform dynamic stretches to warm up your muscles. Dynamic stretching involves active movements that mimic the motions of the exercises you'll be doing during your cardio session. It helps increase body temperature, improve joint mobility, and prepare your muscles for the upcoming activity. Examples of dynamic stretches include leg swings, arm circles, walking lunges, and high knees.

2. Cardiovascular Exercise: Engage in your chosen cardiovascular activity, such as running, cycling,

swimming, or aerobics. Aim to raise your heart rate and maintain a moderate to intense level of activity for the duration of your workout. Depending on your fitness goals, perform cardio exercises for at least 20-30 minutes, or longer if you prefer.

3. Cool Down with Static Stretches: After your cardiovascular workout, take a few minutes to cool down and stretch your muscles. Cool-down stretches are static stretches that help relax the muscles, reduce muscle soreness, and enhance flexibility. Hold each static stretch for about 15-30 seconds, focusing on the major muscle groups used during your cardio workout. Examples of cool-down stretches include standing calf stretches,

seated forward bends, and quad stretches.

4. Post-Workout Stretching: Consider incorporating a more extensive stretching routine after your cardio session, targeting all major muscle groups. This post-workout stretching session can be more focused on improving flexibility and reducing muscle tension. You can include a mix of static stretches, PNF stretching, and foam rolling to aid in muscle recovery and relaxation.

5. Listen to Your Body: Pay attention to how your body feels during and after stretching. Avoid overstretching or forcing yourself into uncomfortable positions. Stretch to the point of mild tension, and if you experience any pain, modify the stretches or

consult with a fitness professional or physical therapist.

6. Make Stretching a Habit: Consistency is key to seeing improvements in flexibility. Aim to stretch regularly, both before and after your cardiovascular workouts. Consider setting aside specific time slots for stretching, such as dedicating 5-10 minutes for dynamic warm-up stretches and another 10-15 minutes for post-workout cool-down and static stretches.

7. Mix It Up: Vary your stretching routine and cardio exercises to keep your fitness routine interesting and challenging. Experiment with different types of stretches and cardio activities to target various muscle groups and prevent workout plateaus.

By incorporating stretching into your cardiovascular exercise routine, you can optimize your fitness efforts, reduce the risk of injuries, and enhance your overall performance and well-being. Remember to customize your stretching routine based on your fitness level and individual needs, and always consult with a healthcare professional or fitness expert if you have any specific concerns or medical conditions.

6.2 Stretching for Strength Training

Stretching is an essential component of a well-rounded strength training routine. Incorporating stretching exercises can improve flexibility, joint mobility, and muscle recovery, leading to better overall performance and reduced risk of injuries. Here's how to effectively include stretching in your strength training workouts:

1. Warm-up with Dynamic Stretches: Begin your strength training session with dynamic stretches to warm up your muscles and prepare them for the upcoming exercises. Dynamic stretching helps increase blood flow, enhance flexibility, and activate the muscles you'll be targeting during your workout. Perform exercises like leg swings, arm circles, hip circles, and bodyweight lunges.

2. Stretch Between Sets: Consider incorporating short static stretches during rest periods between sets. Target the muscles you have just worked on to maintain flexibility and reduce muscle tension. However, avoid holding stretches

for too long, as it may impact your strength performance during the workout.

3. Stretch Targeted Muscle Groups: Focus on stretching the specific muscle groups you have trained during your strength workout. For example, if you did squats or leg exercises, include stretches for the quadriceps, hamstrings, and hip flexors. If you worked on your upper body, include stretches for the chest, shoulders, and back muscles.

4. Utilize PNF Stretching: Proprioceptive Neuromuscular Facilitation (PNF) stretching can be beneficial after your strength training session. PNF stretching involves contracting the targeted muscle before stretching it, which can lead to increased flexibility

and muscle relaxation. For example, perform a partner-assisted hamstring stretch, where you contract your hamstring against resistance before deepening the stretch.

5. Cool-Down with Static Stretches: After completing your strength training routine, dedicate a few minutes to cool down with static stretches. Hold each stretch for about 15-30 seconds to relax the muscles and improve flexibility. Focus on major muscle groups like the quadriceps, hamstrings, calves, chest, shoulders, and back.

6. Foam Rolling: Consider incorporating foam rolling (self-myofascial release) into your post-workout routine. Foam rolling can help release muscle knots and reduce muscle tightness, aiding in

muscle recovery and overall flexibility.

7. Listen to Your Body: Be mindful of your body's signals during stretching. Avoid overstretching or pushing yourself too far, especially after an intense strength training session. Stretch to the point of mild tension and discomfort, but not pain.

6.3 Stretching for Yoga and Pilates

Yoga and Pilates are exercise modalities that naturally incorporate stretching as a fundamental aspect of their practice. Both practices focus on improving flexibility, strength, balance, and body awareness. Here's how stretching is integrated into yoga and Pilates:

1. Dynamic Warm-Up: Yoga and Pilates sessions usually start with a dynamic warm-up that involves flowing movements to gently warm up the body and prepare it for the upcoming static stretches and exercises.

2. Holding Static Stretches: In both yoga and Pilates, various static stretches are held for an extended period, allowing the muscles to lengthen, and the joints to improve their range of motion. Yogic poses (asanas) and Pilates exercises are designed to engage specific muscle groups while stretching others.

3. Mindful Breathing: Breathwork is an integral part of both yoga and Pilates. Deep and mindful

breathing helps practitioners stay present during stretches, relax into the poses, and promote relaxation.

4. Sequencing and Flow: Yoga classes often involve sequences of poses that flow from one to another, combining stretching, strengthening, and balance elements. Pilates exercises are often sequenced to target different muscle groups effectively.

5. Balance and Core Strengthening: In addition to stretching, yoga and Pilates emphasize core strengthening and balance exercises, which complement the overall practice and help with stability during stretching.

6. Modifications: Both yoga and Pilates offer modifications for various poses and exercises,

making them accessible to practitioners of different fitness levels and abilities.

7. Savasana or Final Relaxation: At the end of a yoga session, practitioners typically enjoy savasana, a relaxation pose that allows the body to rest and absorb the benefits of the practice fully. Pilates classes may end with a similar relaxation phase.

8. Regular Practice: Consistent practice is key to experiencing the full benefits of yoga and Pilates. Regularly attending classes or following online tutorials will lead to improved flexibility, strength, and overall well-being.

Yoga and Pilates are practices that encourage self-awareness and self-compassion. Respect your body's limitations and progress at your own pace. Seek guidance from certified yoga instructors or Pilates instructors, especially if you are new to these practices or have specific health concerns. Enjoy the journey of exploration and growth as you incorporate stretching into your yoga and Pilates routines.

6.4 Integrating Stretching into Daily Life

Integrating stretching into your daily life can be a powerful way to improve flexibility, reduce muscle tension, and promote overall well-being. Here are some practical tips to make stretching a natural part of your daily routine:

1. Morning Stretch Routine: Start your day with a few minutes of

gentle stretching. Perform simple stretches for your neck, shoulders, back, and legs to wake up your body and prepare it for the day ahead.

2. Stretch Breaks at Work: Take short stretching breaks throughout your workday. Stand up from your desk and stretch your arms, legs, and back to release tension and improve circulation.

3. Stretch While Watching TV: Utilize commercial breaks or pause your favorite show to do some stretches. Stretch your legs, hips, and spine while enjoying your entertainment.

4. Stretch Before Bed: Incorporate a calming stretching routine before bedtime to relax your body and mind. Focus on gentle stretches

that promote relaxation and help you unwind.

5. Stretch After Physical Activities: Whether you've been sitting at your desk or engaged in physical activities, take a few minutes to stretch afterwards. This can help prevent stiffness and reduce post-activity muscle soreness.

6. Stretch While Waiting: Use waiting times, such as standing in line or waiting for transportation, to do some simple stretches. Stretch your calves, hamstrings, or perform shoulder rolls while waiting.

7. Incorporate Yoga or Pilates: Join a yoga or Pilates class, or follow online tutorials, to integrate guided stretching into your routine. These practices provide a structured and

holistic approach to stretching and overall well-being.

8. Use Stretching Apps: Install stretching apps on your phone or tablet to receive reminders and follow guided stretching routines. Some apps offer customizable routines tailored to your needs and fitness level.

9. Mindful Stretching: Approach stretching with mindfulness and focus on your breath and body sensations. Be present and fully engage with each stretch to maximize its benefits.

10. Set Stretching Goals: Set realistic stretching goals for yourself, such as aiming to stretch for 10 minutes every morning or including specific stretches to target areas of tightness.

11. Stretch with a Partner: Engage in partner stretching sessions with a friend or family member. Partner stretching can deepen the stretches and create a sense of accountability and camaraderie.

12. Make It Fun: Make stretching enjoyable by incorporating music or trying different stretching styles like dance-inspired stretches or animal-inspired movements.

Consistency is key when integrating stretching into your daily life. Small, regular stretching sessions can lead to significant improvements in flexibility and overall mobility. Be kind to yourself and listen to your body; never force stretches or push beyond your limits. If you have any specific health concerns, consider consulting with a healthcare professional or fitness expert before starting a new stretching routine. Enjoy the process of incorporating stretching into your daily life and experience the positive impact it can have on your overall well-being.

www.ingramcontent.com/pod-product-compliance
Lightning Source LLC
Chambersburg PA
CBHW070912260726
48661CB00004B/1709